ANATOMY OF FITNESS™

Yoga

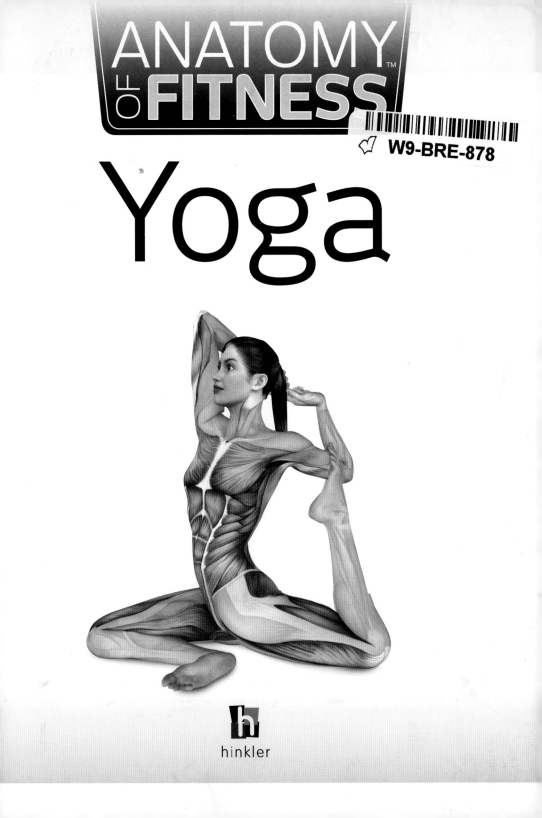

hinkler

Published by Hinkler Books Pty Ltd 2012
45–55 Fairchild Street
Heatherton Victoria 3202 Australia
www.hinkler.com.au

hinkler

Copyright © Hinkler Books Pty Ltd 2012

Created by Moseley Road Inc.
Editorial director: Lisa Purcell
Art director: Brian MacMullen
Cover and internals designer: Sam Grimmer
Photographer: Jonathan Conklin Photography, Inc.
Author: Goldie Karpel Oren
Model: Lana Russo
Illustrator: Hector Aiza/3DLabz
Prepress: Graphic Print Group
Inset illustrations © Linda Bucklin/Shutterstock.com,
page 5 © heaven/Shutterstock.com,
page 6 © Ekaterina Garyuk/Shutterstock.com,
page 7 top © Brooke Becker/Shutterstock.com,
page 7 bottom © StockLite/Shutterstock.com,
page 9 © zhuda/Shutterstock.com

ISBN: 978 1 7430 8740 4

Printed and bound in China

Always do the warm-up exercises before attempting any individual exercises. It is recommended that you check with
your doctor or healthcare professional before commencing any exercise regime. While every care has been taken in
the preparation of this material, the publishers and their respective employees or agents will not accept responsibility
for injury or damage occasioned to any person as a result of participation in the activities described in this book.

Contents

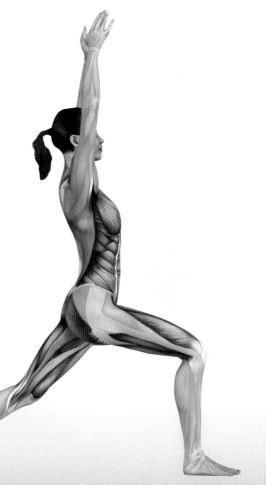

Yoga: Mind & Body Fitness

The practice of yoga not only disciplines your body, but also helps to discipline your mind.

Yoga is more than just another form of fitness: the practice transcends the physicality of its postures. Yoga is also a mental and spiritual practice, in the sense that the work that goes into aligning the body can also be used to align your mind.

In yoga we are trying to calm the fluctuations of the mind. Our minds have a tendency to think in past and future tenses. In yoga, we have to concentrate on keeping our thoughts in the present moment. You will find, by practicing this technique, that you are more fully present on a daily basis.

This book contains a well-balanced, flowing sequence of poses. You will build strength and flexibility while improving your concentration and willpower. You will learn to control your body with your mind and come to understand that, as in life, with time and patience you can overcome many obstacles.

You will see, for example, that your mind will want to give up before your body needs to come out of a pose; you'll learn to understand the distinction between pain and discomfort. If you suffer actual pain from an injury then you should come out of a pose, but otherwise, try to breathe through any discomfort.

Sometimes you will have intense sensations in your muscles—it is normal to have these feelings while holding a yoga pose. Sometimes we have to ignore what our minds are telling us and move beyond thinking, "I can't hold this any longer." *Your body is strong enough to hold the posture for longer than you think. By holding a yoga pose for a*

Challenge yourself

Your breath will get you through the demanding poses. For instance, challenge yourself to hold Plank Pose (pages 28–29) for one or even two minutes, which is about 10 to 20 long, deep breath cycles. Not only will you build core strength, but you will also cultivate internal strength, stamina, and willpower. Stay in the position longer than you want to. Finding stillness of the body and stillness of the mind is the most challenging aspect of yoga. Holding the poses is often more difficult than moving and flowing.

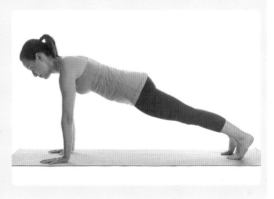

few extra breaths, you will begin to build inner strength. You will learn that you are stronger than you imagined.

In the world we live in, we are used to instant gratification. By practicing yoga and holding the poses, which can be uncomfortable, you will build patience. You will find that you can take a step back, pause, and breathe. You will find that turning off your phone for an hour and rolling out your mat can be quite rewarding. You will know, when you finish with your practice, that you can take an hour to shut out your to-do lists and distracting thoughts, following through on an important decision to focus on your breath and the alignment of your body.

You will be able to use lessons learned on the yoga mat in your daily life, knowing that no challenging situation will last forever, just as no yoga posture lasts forever. Yoga teaches us to be completely present in every moment of our lives, whether it is

a good time or a bad one. Stress is often brought on by worrying about the future, or by dwelling on events in the past. The stress that you experience may be caused by the thoughts in your head—the situation you are in may not actually be too stressful after all. With your yoga practice, you will see that by changing how you think about things, you can change your outlook. So give yourself that extra moment to pause and take a deep breath.

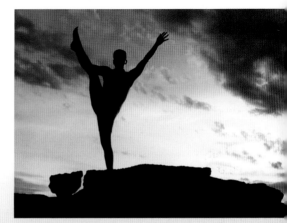

Home Practice

To get the most out of your yoga practice, dedicate a
particular area within your home as your yoga space.
This is where you should practice on a regular schedule.

The greatest challenge of practicing
yoga at home, rather than at a
studio, is learning to shut out all
potential distractions. Your family, phones,
computer, and television can prevent
you from concentrating on what you are
doing. When practicing at home, you need
to create a space in which you can block
out those distractions. Designate a room
or area where you will always practice.
Make a schedule for yourself, setting
aside perhaps 30 minutes at the same
time every day, five days a week. The
great thing about yoga is that you don't
need a lot of space—just the length of the
yoga mat. When traveling, you can pack
your mat in your suitcase and roll it out
wherever you are.

Equipment and clothing

To begin your home practice, you will need
a yoga block, a yoga strap, and a yoga
mat. A block aids you during standing
poses that call for you to place a hand on
the floor. A strap helps you to achieve a
full stretch. And you don't need specially
designed yoga equipment: a book will
easily stand in for a yoga block, and a
long belt or sash will work just as well as
a yoga strap. A yoga mat is different from
a Pilates mat or a padded gym mat. Buy
a mat specifically designed for yoga that
is thin and sticky, so that you have the
traction to grip the floor with your hands
and feet. Wear a comfortable top and
pants, and leave off the socks. Practicing
barefoot will help you to ground your
hands and feet into the floor.

Flexibility and body awareness

Everyone has a different level of natural
flexibility; strength and flexibility are two
traits that, as humans, we need to work
on constantly. Don't feel that you
can't take a yoga class because
you're not flexible! This is why
we call yoga a "practice."
Each individual has a
tendency toward either being
more flexible or having tighter
muscles, and in yoga we're trying to
find that balance between our strength

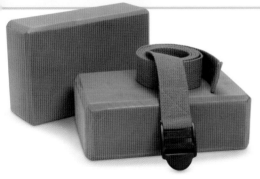

and our flexibility. Our bodies and minds are constantly changing and evolving—every time you come to your mat you will feel different than you felt the last time you did yoga. This is what makes the yoga practice interesting. We may perform the same poses time and time again, yet each time we find something new to work on. An advanced practitioner is not necessarily someone who can come into the most challenging pose; being advanced means having the body awareness and control to work the subtleties of each pose.

Using your tools

Think of your yoga props as tools to help you deepen your poses. Don't think that using the block and strap makes you a "beginner," or that you're not really doing the pose if you use them. In Extended Triangle with Block (pages 36–37), for example, the point of the pose is not to reach your palms to the floor; the goal is to elongate your spine, finding length on all four sides of your torso. If your hand is on the floor but the side of your body is crunched and you can't breathe, then you're not doing yoga—you are just contorting your body. Instead, use your block to your advantage, and create the space you need to deepen your breath.

Dedicated space

There's no need to call in a carpenter to build you a home yoga studio. Your goal is to simply reserve a quiet space within your home—a space in which to retreat regularly to practice yoga.

If you live in a large house, you may have the luxury of transforming an entire room into a private yoga studio. But if your space is smaller, you can still create a peaceful sanctuary. Just designate an area large enough to stretch fully and lunge freely, without obstructions. A movable screen, such as a folding Shoji screen, can lend privacy, as can curtains or drapery that you can easily open and close.

Store your yoga mat, blocks, straps, and other gear within this space for easy access, and don't forget the atmosphere-setting extras. Gather things that inspire you: plants, stones, and other natural objects can set the mood. A swirling image that you can meditate on or a flickering candle for your eyes to lock onto while you hold that pose just a few breaths longer can add greatly to your yoga practice.

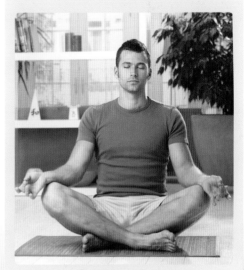

Breath Control

We may take breathing—the very essence of life—for granted, but learning how to do it properly and mindfully will enhance your yoga practice.

Your breath will guide you through your practice. The style of the sequence in this book is that of a Vinyasa flow class. The word *vinyasa* means "to link" or "to connect." In your practice you are linking your breath with your movement, and your movement with your breath. You will

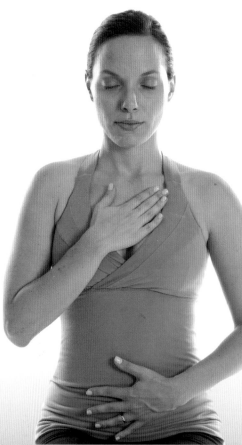

begin to create a moving meditation. As you hold the poses and flow from one to the next, you'll focus on lengthening and·deepening your breath, and in this way yoga is simply a breathing exercise. If you find yourself holding your breath or breathing heavily, take a step back and re-evaluate your position. This may mean holding the pose for a shorter time, choosing a less challenging variation of the posture, or resting in Child's Pose (pages 14–15). Our minds constantly jump from thought to thought, focusing on situations and stories from the past and worrying about and planning the future, so that much of the time we forget to live in the present moment. The breath is our tool for staying in the present moment. By concentrating on our breath, we are forced to put aside any other thoughts that may be cluttering up our brains.

Pranayama

In Sanskrit, *prana* means "life force" or "energy," and *ayama* means "to control or extend." Together the two form the word *pranayama*, which means "extension of the life force," or "breath control." The practice of yoga calls for us to pay close attention to the process of breathing in and out, which we usually take for granted.

Kapalabhati

There are several ways to manipulate the breath. One of the most common methods of warm-up breathing is Kapalabhati. *Kapal* means "skull," and *bhati* means "shining"; together the two words mean "shining skull." This is a breathing technique that will cleanse your sinuses. In Kapalabhati, you control the breath by sharply exhaling while pumping your stomach in and out. The inhalation is passive, while the exhalation is forceful and sharp. The sharp and rapid exhales will help your lungs to clear any waste from your air passageways.

Ujjayi Pranayama

Another common breathing technique is Ujjayi Pranayama. This technique calms the brain and creates internal heat. When done correctly, Ujjayi sounds like the ocean, so it is often called "ocean breath." During the execution of Ujjayi Pranayama, your mouth stays closed, and there is a slight constriction of your throat as you inhale and exhale.

Because it is deep and mindful, the breath will help to calm your nervous system. This type of breath will help to reduce stress by stimulating the parasympathetic response of the central nervous system instead of the fight-or-flight response, which increases adrenaline. This relaxation response will help to quiet your mind, reduce stress, and make you feel good when you leave your mat.

Practicing Ujjayi
Proper breath is an essential element of yoga. Start by practicing Ujjayi Pranayama.

1 Begin by sitting up tall in a comfortable position, such as Easy Pose (pages 12–13).

2 Hold your hand in front of your mouth and imagine that your hand is a mirror. Open your mouth and exhale a *hah* sound, as if you were fogging up a mirror. That breath comes from the back of your throat.

3 Now close your mouth, and try to breathe in a similar way, as if you were fogging up that imaginary mirror. You will notice a hissing sound coming from the back of your throat. This is the start to practicing the Ujjayi breathing technique.

Practice about 8 to 10 breath cycles, inhaling and exhaling with this slight constriction at the back of your throat. As you begin to feel more comfortable, you will naturally start to breathe in this way throughout the entire vinyasa yoga practice. The Ujjayi technique will start to effortlessly flow from one breath to the next, helping you to connect your movement with your breath.

The Yoga Sequence

The following pages will guide you through a flowing sequence of poses that help to increase strength and flexibility while improving concentration and willpower.

The yoga sequence in this book consists of 24 individual yoga poses. Some of the poses will be repeated. For each pose, you will find step-by-step instructions as well as notes on correct form. You can make the practice your own by going at your own pace; if you like, you can stay in the poses longer than recommended, taking extra breaths where you need to.

How to practice the yoga sequence

Begin the yoga sequence by taking a seated position, with your eyes closed. Use this time to center yourself and bring your awareness to your breath.

From the seated position you will make your way into Downward-Facing Dog, a pose that you will come into often throughout the flow. You will go on to perform several Sun Salutation A's to build internal heat as you warm up. The Sun Salutations help you connect to your breath. The flowing sequence focuses the mind and synchronizes it with your body and breath, drawing you deeper into the practice. Each pose that forms part of the Sun Salutation A sequence is connected to a breath call, either an inhalation or an exhalation. The sequence flows smoothly from pose to pose, using the breath to help move you.

Terms to know

Certain terms that are often heard in a yoga class will appear throughout the book.

vinyasa: The word *vinyasa* literally means "to link or connect." In a yoga class it can also mean a specific sequence of breath-synchronized movements used to transition between sustained postures: Plank Pose, Chaturanga, Upward-Facing Dog, Downward-Facing Dog. The entire sequence of poses in this book can also be called "vinyasa" because you are linking your breath with your movement and your movement with your breath.

alignment: In the yoga practice each pose has an ideal position of the body. If the body is in alignment, then it is placed in a proper way so that the muscles can work more effectively; they don't have to grip or struggle to hold the position, thus preventing injury. Each pose has its own alignment points, such as where to place your hands, feet, or torso, so learning a pose means also learning its proper points of alignment.

heel-to-heel alignment: When your feet are separated wide apart, if you were draw a line from one foot to the other, the heels would be on the same line. This type of alignment is used when practicing internally rotated postures.

heel-to-arch alignment: When your feet are separated wide apart, if you were draw a line from your front foot, it would intersect with the inner arch of the back foot. This type of alignment is used in externally rotated postures.

internally rotate: The body part moves in toward the center of the body.

externally rotate: The body part moves away from the center of the body.

ground down: To press your hands or feet (foundation) into the floor.

energy up: Energy isn't tangible, but in the yoga practice you are moving stale energy around and trying to lift your energy levels. "Energy up" is a subtle feeling of an upward lift.

After Sun Salutation A you will hold several externally rotated standing positions, which will help to open your hips. Next, you will move into the internally rotated postures that form Sun Salutation B, either choosing to hold Chair or Warrior I, or flow through the sequence holding each pose in the sequence for one breath. After the standing postures you will practice backbends, often called "heart-openers." You'll then begin to cool down and calm your mind with several stretches and forward bends leading up to your final deep relaxation, called Savasana, or Corpse Pose.

DVD section 2: Chapter 1

Easy Pose
(Sukhasana)

If your hamstrings, lower back, or hip flexors are tight then Easy Pose will not be so easy! As you continue to practice yoga, you will find the pose becoming more comfortable—and in time, you'll be able to sit and meditate for hours.

1 Sit on the floor, bend your knees, and cross your legs at the shins. Flex your feet to keep your knees in alignment. Feel both sitting bones firmly pressing into the floor and find a neutral pelvis. Lengthen your spine by sitting up straight and opening up across your collarbones.

2 Place your hands on your thighs with your palms facing either up or down.

3 Close your eyes and draw your focus inward. Lengthen your inhalation and exhalation, aiming for equal length. Try to match the length of your exhale to your inhale. Hold this pose for 5 to 10 breaths.

4 Easy Pose is a common position used for Pranayama and meditation. Close your eyes and draw your focus inward. You can begin by simply lengthening your inhalation and lengthening your exhalation. Try to match the length of your exhale to your inhale. Hold this pose for 1 to 3 minutes.

Diary of practice

	Date	No. of Breaths	Comment
Week 1			
Week 2			
Week 3			
Week 4			

Correct form

· Sit on a block or blanket to elevate your hips above the level of your knees.
· Alternate the crossing of your shins. We all have a dominant side; allow your less dominant side to stretch and find balance in the hips by switching the crossing of your shins.

Avoid

· Letting your knees rise above your hips.
· Rounding your shoulders.

Annotation Key
* indicates deep muscles

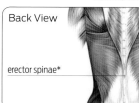

Back View

erector spinae*

gluteus medius*

rectus abdominis

iliopsoas*

sartorius

transversus abdominis*

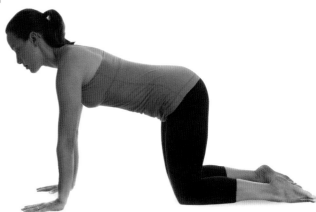

Child's Pose

(Balasana)

Very relaxing and restorative, Child's Pose is a perfect resting position that you can assume at any point during your practice.

1 From Easy Pose (pages 12–13), uncross your legs and come onto your hands and knees.

2 Bring your big toes together and your knees about hip-distance apart.

3 Sit your hips back onto your heels as you extend your torso forward, laying your stomach onto your thighs. Let your shoulders round forward, allowing your forehead to rest gently on the floor.

4 Bring your arms by your sides with the palms of your hands facing upward. Breathe into the back of your body. Hold for 5 to 10 breaths.

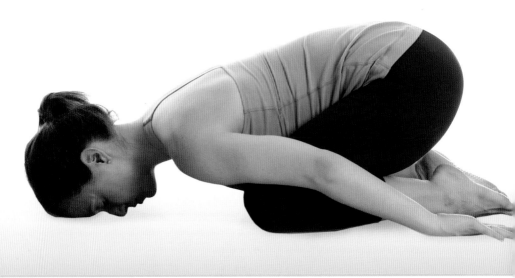

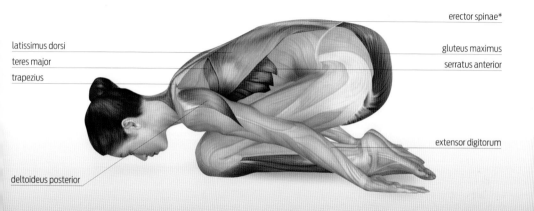

Diary of practice

	Date	No. of Breaths	Comment
Week 1			
Week 2			
Week 3			
Week 4			

Correct form
· Relax any tension you are holding in your jaw and face muscles.
· Open up between your shoulder blades as you breathe.

Avoid
· Bringing your knees too far apart.

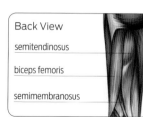

Front View

tibialis anterior

peroneus

Back View

semitendinosus

biceps femoris

semimembranosus

Annotation Key
* indicates deep muscles

erector spinae*

latissimus dorsi

teres major

trapezius

gluteus maximus

serratus anterior

extensor digitorum

deltoideus posterior

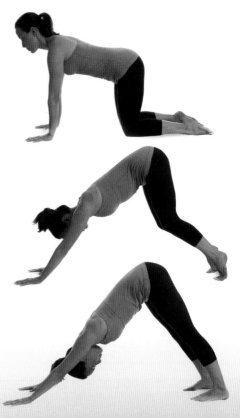

Downward-Facing Dog
(Adho Mukha Svanasana)

Downward-Facing Dog is among the most frequently performed yoga poses—one you'll come into time and again. "Down Dog," as it is often known, stretches and strengthens the entire body. Because your head is below your heart in this pose, it is known as an "inversion."

1 From Child's Pose (pages 14–15), come onto your hands and knees, with your hands aligned under your shoulders and your knees under your hips.

2 Tuck your toes under, and "walk" your hands forward about a palm's distance in front of your shoulders. With hands and toes planted, lift your hips up as you straighten your legs and draw your heels toward the floor.

3 Press your chest toward your thighs, and bring your head between your arms. Lengthen up through your tailbone and keep your thighs slightly internally rotated, finding a neutral pelvis. Gaze between your feet or toward your navel. Hold for 5 to 10 breaths.

Correct form
- If you have tight shoulders, plant your hands more widely, and if the backs of your legs are tight, plant your feet more widely.
- To find the correct foot position, lift your toes, spread them out, and lower them. Press evenly through your feet and draw your inner ankles up to lift your arches, and then bring your heels toward the floor.
- To focus on your arms and hands, line up your wrist creases parallel to the front of the mat, resist your forearms away from the floor, and externally rotate your outer upper arms, drawing your inner elbows forward. Spread your fingers wide and ground down through every knuckle. Keep your middle finger pointing forward.

Avoid
- Internally rotating your arms and sinking into your shoulders.
- Rounding or over-arching your lower back.
- Letting your front ribs jut forward.

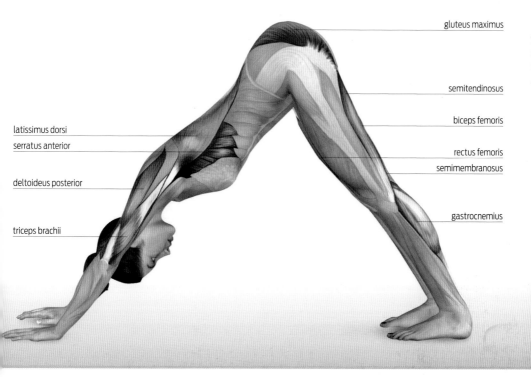

Diary of practice

	Date	No. of Breaths	Comment
Week 1			
Week 2			
Week 3			
Week 4			

gluteus maximus

semitendinosus

biceps femoris

rectus femoris
semimembranosus

gastrocnemius

latissimus dorsi

serratus anterior

deltoideus posterior

triceps brachii

High Lunge

High Lunge is a pose that can be held for several breaths or used as a transitional pose in the Sun Salutation sequences as a way to step back to Downward-Facing Dog or as a way to step forward into Standing Forward Bend.

1 From Downward-Facing Dog (pages 16–17), step your left foot forward in between your hands, with your left knee and shin lined up over your left ankle.

2 With your fingertips resting on the floor, square your hips to the front of the mat, grounding your left heel into the floor and drawing your left hip crease back.

3 Extend your right leg straight behind you, resting the ball of your foot on the mat. Lengthen all the way from the crown of your head to your right heel. Gaze slightly ahead, keeping the back of your neck long. Hold for 1 to 5 breaths. Later in the sequence, repeat on the other side.

Correct form
- Bring your belly in, away from your thigh.
- Keep your thighs firm as you stretch.
- Roll the inner thigh of your straight leg toward the ceiling, finding its internal rotation.
- If your back begins rounding when your fingertips touch the floor, bring your hands onto blocks to help elongate your spine.

Avoid
- Letting your stomach hang down.
- Positioning your knee past your ankle and over your toes, which can stress your knee joint.

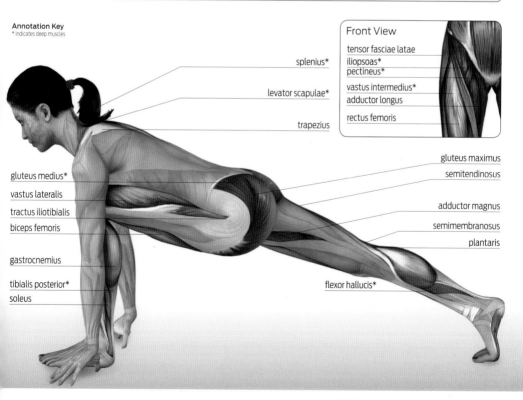

Diary of practice

	Date	No. of Breaths	Comment
Week 1			
Week 2			
Week 3			
Week 4			

Annotation Key
* indicates deep muscles

splenius*

levator scapulae*

trapezius

Front View

tensor fasciae latae
iliopsoas*
pectineus*

vastus intermedius*
adductor longus

rectus femoris

gluteus medius*

vastus lateralis

tractus iliotibialis

biceps femoris

gastrocnemius

tibialis posterior*

soleus

gluteus maximus

semitendinosus

adductor magnus

semimembranosus

plantaris

flexor hallucis*

Standing Half Forward Bend to Standing Forward Bend
(Ardha Uttanasana to Uttanasana)

Often repeated throughout yoga classes, Standing Half Forward Bend and Standing Forward Bend form part of the Sun Salutation sequences. Each time you perform these poses, you will fold a little deeper into the forward bend.

1 From High Lunge (pages 18–19), inhale to step your back foot forward to meet your front foot. Spread out your toes and press down evenly through all four corners of your feet.

2 Plant your fingertips in line with your toes and look forward. Straighten your legs and arms as you lift your chest up away from your legs. Broaden across the front of your chest, finding a slight backward bend in your upper back as you draw your stomach in.

3 Press your heels into the floor as you lift your tailbone up toward the ceiling, keeping your hips in line with your heels. This is Standing Half Forward Bend.

4 Inhale to lengthen your spine, then exhale as you fold forward, hinging at the hips and bringing your fingertips or palms to the floor. This is Standing Forward Bend.

5 Lengthen your torso as you bring your belly closer to your thighs, ground your heels into the floor, and lift your tailbone toward the ceiling. Hold for 1 to 5 breaths, inhaling to lengthen the spine and exhaling to fold deeper.

Correct form
- Keep a slight bend in your knees if you have a tight lower back or hamstrings. Separating your feet hip-width apart also helps if you have tight hamstrings.
- If you can't reach the floor during Standing Half Forward Bend, place your hands on your shins.
- If you cannot reach the floor during Standing Forward Bend, place your hands on blocks or bend your arms and hold opposite elbows.

Avoid
- Shifting your weight backward so that your hips are behind your heels.

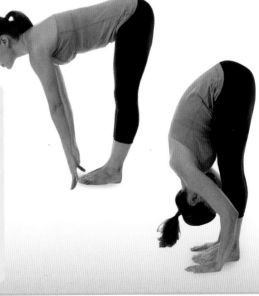

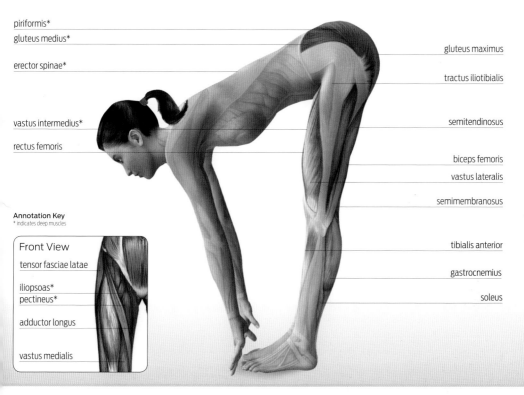

Diary of practice

	Date	No. of Breaths	Comment
Week 1			
Week 2			
Week 3			
Week 4			

piriformis*

gluteus medius*

erector spinae*

gluteus maximus

tractus iliotibialis

vastus intermedius*

semitendinosus

rectus femoris

biceps femoris

vastus lateralis

semimembranosus

Annotation Key
* indicates deep muscles

tibialis anterior

gastrocnemius

soleus

Front View

tensor fasciae latae

iliopsoas*
pectineus*

adductor longus

vastus medialis

Upward Salute
(Urdhva Hastasana)

Upward Salute is the second pose in the Sun Salutation A series. In the traditional posture, the arms are separated; if your shoulders are more open, you can join your hands together above your head while keeping your arms straight.

1 From Standing Forward Bend (pages 20–21), inhale as you lift your torso up, keeping your back flat as you reach your arms out to your sides, and continue lifting until you are standing with your arms above your head. Your hands should be shoulder-width apart.

2 Straighten your arms, and rotate your shoulders externally open so that the palms of your hands face each other, spreading up through the fingertips.

3 Gaze forward or tilt your head slightly back, and bring your gaze up to your thumbs. Hold for 1 to 5 breaths.

Correct form
· Stretch your arms completely straight from your elbows.
· Soften any tension in your shoulders.

Avoid
· Tensing your shoulders up toward your ears.
· Bending your elbows.

Diary of practice

	Date	No. of Breaths	Comment
Week 1			
Week 2			
Week 3			
Week 4			

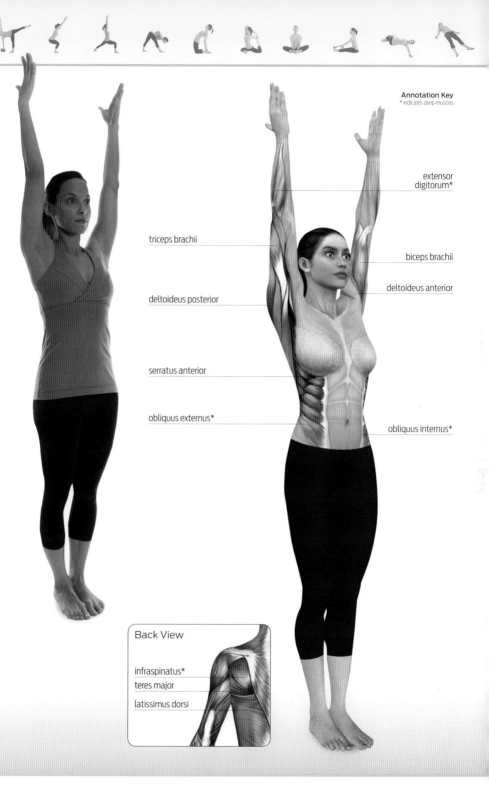

extensor
digitorum*

triceps brachii

biceps brachii

deltoideus posterior

deltoideus anterior

serratus anterior

obliquus externus*

obliquus internus*

Back View

infraspinatus*

teres major

latissimus dorsi

Mountain Pose
(Tadasana)

Mountain Pose is the basis for many standing poses. Although this posture may seem simple, it can actually be quite challenging to achieve the correct alignment.

1 From Upward Salute (pages 22–23), exhale as you bring your arms to your sides. Your feet should be together as you stand tall.

2 Breathe in and out as you maintain the pose. Find your balance, keeping your pelvis neutral by drawing the tip of your tailbone down toward your feet as you lift your hip bones upward. Your weight may shift in a circular motion as you balance. Root and rebound, feeling your feet grounded onto the floor as energy radiates from the feet up through the top of your head.

Diary of practice

	Date	No. of Breaths	Comment
Week 1			
Week 2			
Week 3			
Week 4			

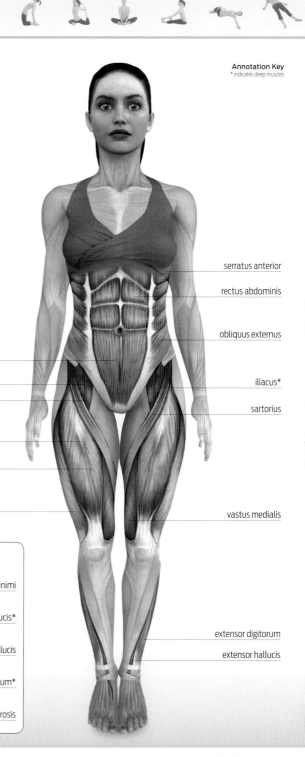

Correct form

- Release any tension in the facial area.
- Stand completely straight with shoulders stacked over hips, hips stacked over knees, and knees in line with feet.
- Visualize your pelvis as a bowl of soup—you don't want to spill it forward or backward.
- Stretch your arms straight, with energy reaching out of your fingertips.
- Keep your chin parallel to the floor, and the crown of your head pressing upward.

Avoid

- Arching your lower back.
- Pushing your ribs forward.
- Over-tucking your pelvis.
- Holding your breath.

serratus anterior

rectus abdominis

obliquus externus

transversus abdominis*

iliopsoas*

pectineus*

iliacus*

sartorius

vastus intermedius*

rectus femoris

vastus lateralis

vastus medialis

extensor digitorum

extensor hallucis

Bottom of Foot

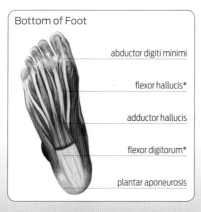

abductor digiti minimi

flexor hallucis*

adductor hallucis

flexor digitorum*

plantar aponeurosis

Tree Pose
(Vrksasana)

In Tree Pose, as your standing foot stays strongly rooted to the floor and the top of your head reaches up toward the ceiling, you will feel energy moving down and up at the same time.

1 From Mountain Pose (pages 24–25), bend your right knee, bringing your foot up to your left inner thigh, with toes pointing to the floor.

2 Externally rotate your right thigh, allowing your right knee to point out to the right while keeping your hips level.

3 Continue to open your right hip, rotating your inner thigh clockwise as you draw your tailbone down toward your left heel to neutralize your

pelvis. Press your right foot into your left inner thigh as you draw your left outer hip in for stability.

4 Find your balance, and then join your hands in a prayer position. Hold for 1 to 5 breaths.

5 Release your right foot back down into Mountain Pose (pages 24–25), and repeat the pose on the other leg. Stand in Mountain Pose when finished to begin the Sun Salutation A sequence (page 60).

Diary of practice

	Date	No. of Breaths	Comment
Week 1			
Week 2			
Week 3			
Week 4			

Correct form

- Keep your standing leg in place with the foot facing straight ahead. Ground down through all four corners of this foot to help you balance throughout the exercise.
- If you need help placing your foot at your thigh, grasp the ankle with your hand.
- If you have trouble bringing your foot all the way up to your inner thigh, rest it on the side of your shin instead.
- To assist in balancing, place your heel at your ankle with the ball of the foot on the floor, or lean against a wall.

Avoid

- Resting your foot on the sensitive kneecap area.

transversus abdominis*

rectus abdominis

obliquus externus

iliopsoas*

iliacus*
pectineus*

obliquus internus*

tensor fasciae latae

adductor longus

sartorius

vastus intermedius*

rectus femoris

gracilis

vastus lateralis

vastus medialis

gastrocnemius

tibialis anterior

soleus

Back View

quadratus lumborum*

gluteus medius*

gluteus maximus

quadratus femoris*

obdurator internus*

obdurator externus*

Plank Pose

Plank Pose is part of the traditional Sun Salutation sequence, as well as the vinyasa that you will repeat several times throughout this yoga sequence. This vinyasa consists of Plank Pose, Chaturanga, Upward-Facing Dog, and Downward-Facing Dog. Plank can also be practiced on its own. Challenge yourself by holding it for 30 seconds, 1 minute, or eventually even 2 or 3 minutes.

1 From High Lunge (pages 18–19), place your hands flat on the floor and step your front foot backward to meet your back foot.

2 Inhale, and shift your weight forward so that your shoulders are in line with your wrists. Come onto the balls of your feet with your toes spread out and your heels reaching back. Keep your arms straight and parallel to each other, externally rotating your outer upper arms so that your inner elbows draw forward. As you hold the pose, soften between your shoulder blades and melt your heart down as you broaden across the collarbones to lift your sternum. Internally rotate your inner thighs, keeping the thighs firm. Lengthen your tailbone down toward your heels. Hold for 1 to 5 breaths.

Correct form
· Make sure that your wrist creases are parallel to the front of the mat.
· Spread your fingers wide, and ground down through every knuckle.
· Use your breath to get you through holding the pose.

Avoid
· Lifting your fingers off the floor.
· Rounding your upper back.

Diary of practice

	Date	No. of Breaths	Comment
Week 1			
Week 2			
Week 3			
Week 4			

Annotation Key
* indicates deep muscles

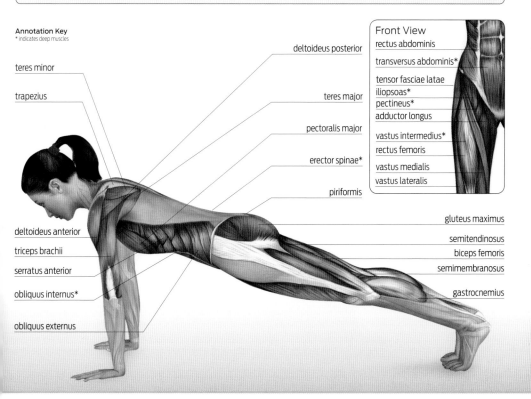

deltoideus posterior

teres minor

trapezius

teres major

pectoralis major

erector spinae*

piriformis

Front View
rectus abdominis
transversus abdominis*
tensor fasciae latae
iliopsoas*
pectineus*
adductor longus
vastus intermedius*
rectus femoris
vastus medialis
vastus lateralis

gluteus maximus
semitendinosus
biceps femoris
semimembranosus
gastrocnemius

deltoideus anterior
triceps brachii
serratus anterior
obliquus internus*
obliquus externus

Chaturanga
(Chaturanga Dandasana)

Chaturanga, sometimes called Four-Limbed Staff Pose, is practiced in Sun Salutation A and B. It is also part of the vinyasa shown on page 62. Like Plank Pose, Chaturanga challenges your core strength and stability.

1 From Plank Pose (pages 28–29), shift your weight forward toward the tips of your toes. Exhale as you bend your elbows over your wrists and lower yourself down so that your shoulders are in line with your elbows. As you lower, ground your palm and fingers down into the floor. The thumb and index finger have a tendency to want to lift up, so make a special effort to press down between the two.

2 Hold the pose, rotating your inner thighs and drawing your tailbone downward so that you don't sink into your lower back. Lift your thighs away from the floor. Draw your shoulder blades together as you lift the heads of the shoulders away from the floor.

Correct form
· Keep the back of your neck long by gazing slightly beyond the edge of your mat.

Avoid
· Bending your elbows so much that your chest collapses and your shoulders round forward.
· Dropping hips lower than your shoulders.

Diary of practice

	Date	No. of Breaths	Comment
Week 1			
Week 2			
Week 3			
Week 4			

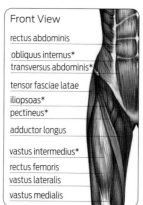

gluteus maximus

triceps brachii

teres minor

deltoideus posterior

pectoralis major

serratus anterior

obliquus externus

Front View

rectus abdominis

obliquus internus*

transversus abdominis*

tensor fasciae latae

iliopsoas*

pectineus*

adductor longus

vastus intermedius*

rectus femoris

vastus lateralis

vastus medialis

Annotation Key
* indicates deep muscles

semitendinosus

biceps femoris

semimembranosus

gastrocnemius

soleus

Upward-Facing Dog
(Urdhva Mukha Svanasana)

Upward-Facing Dog is a backbend posture in both of the Sun Salutation sequences. It is also a step in the vinyasa, along with Plank Pose, Chaturanga, and Downward-Facing Dog.

1 From Chaturanga (pages 30–31), inhale and straighten your arms so that your shoulders are directly above your wrists as you flip to the tops of both feet, keeping your thighs and knees off the floor the entire time. Spread your fingers, and ground down. Draw your tailbone down, and lift your pubic bone toward your belly button.

2 To continue the sequence, exhale, lifting your hips up as you simultaneously flip your feet and transition to Downward-Facing Dog. Hold for 1 to 5 breaths.

Correct form
- Keep your wrists parallel to the front edge of your mat, and position your shoulders above your wrists.
- Keep your chin tucked slightly as you lengthen the back of your neck.
- While holding the pose, focus on a comfortable gazing point, such as the spot where wall and ceiling meet.

Avoid
- Resting your thighs on the floor.
- Positioning your hands in front of your shoulders.
- Externally rotating your thighs, as this can compress your lower back.

Diary of practice

	Date	No. of Breaths	Comment
Week 1			
Week 2			
Week 3			
Week 4			

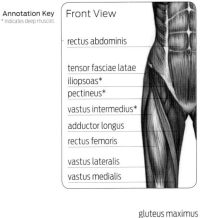

Annotation Key
* indicates deep muscles

Front View

rectus abdominis

tensor fasciae latae
iliopsoas*
pectineus*
vastus intermedius*
adductor longus
rectus femoris
vastus lateralis
vastus medialis

sternocleidomastoideus

teres minor

rhomboideus*

erector spinae*

latissimus dorsi

triceps brachii

gluteus maximus

adductor magnus

semitendinosus

biceps femoris

semimembranosus

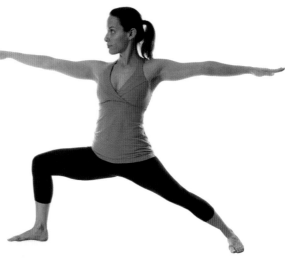

Warrior II
(Virabhadrasana II)

One of the three Warrior poses performed in yoga, Warrior II is often performed earlier in a sequence than Warrior I. Mastering Warrior II will help you build the inner strength and courage of a warrior.

1 From Downward-Facing Dog (pages 16–17), step the right foot forward, to come into High Lunge (pages 18–19).

2 Pivot your left heel down, and turn your foot out 45 degrees. Walk your right foot to the left several inches so that your right heel aligns with the inner arch of your left foot.

3 Keeping your right knee bent, lift your torso so that your shoulders line up over your hips. Keep a slight internal rotation to the back leg to keep the leg neutral. Extend both arms out to the sides, parallel to the floor, with palms facing downward. Continue to bend your right knee so that your thigh is parallel to the floor, externally rotating your right hip to open your thigh. Find a neutral pelvis. Turn your head to the right and gaze past your fingers.

4 Hold for 1 to 5 breaths. Later in the sequence, repeat on the other side.

Correct form
· Press your heels into the floor, using your inner-thigh muscles.
· Keep your shoulders directly above your hips.
· When holding the pose, make sure that your front knee is in line with your middle toe.

Avoid
· Arching your lower back.
· Leaning forward over your bent leg.

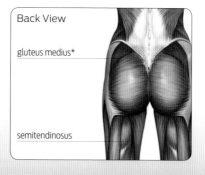

Back View

gluteus medius*

semitendinosus

Diary of practice

	Date	No. of Breaths	Comment
Week 1			
Week 2			
Week 3			
Week 4			

Annotation Key
* indicates deep muscles

scalenus*

sternocleidomastoideus

vastus intermedius*
rectus femoris

vastus
medialis

tensor fasciae latae

adductor longus
biceps femoris
gracilis*
vastus lateralis

Extended Triangle with Block
(Utthita Trikonasana)

Extended Triangle Pose encompasses the entire body. It is a hip opener, core strengthener, side bend, twist, and heart opener. This version allows you to use a yoga block, which means less stress on tight hamstrings and hips.

1 From Warrior II (pages 34–35), inhale to straighten your right leg by firming your thigh and lifting your kneecap upward. You may need to shorten your stance by about 6 to 12 inches (15 to 30 cm). Keep your right heel in line with the center of your left foot. Externally rotate your right thigh while keeping your back leg neutral.

2 Keeping both legs straight with firm thighs and your arms extended out to your sides parallel to the floor, exhale and reach your right arm and torso down to the right as you shift your hips to the left, deepening the crease in your right hip.

3 Place your right hand on the block on the outside of your right leg. Extend your left arm straight up, with fingers spread. Inhale as you find length across your collarbones.

4 Exhale, and turn the right side of your torso toward the ceiling.

5 Inhale as you turn your head to gaze up at your left fingertips. Hold for 1 to 5 breaths. Later in the sequence, repeat on the other side.

Correct form
· Bend from your hips, not from your waist.
· Keep your thighs engaged by maintaining a very slight bend in your knees.
· Stand as if you were in between two panes of glass.
· Position the block directly underneath your shoulder.

Avoid
· Straightening your legs so much that your knees lock.
· Crunching the bottom side of your torso while bending.
· Leaning forward.

Diary of practice

	Date	No. of Breaths	Comment
Week 1			
Week 2			
Week 3			
Week 4			

Back View

latissimus dorsi

quadratus lumborum*

gluteus medius*

gluteus maximus

quadratus femoris*

obdurator internus*
obdurator externus*

semitendinosus

biceps femoris

semimembranosus

Annotation Key
* indicates deep muscles

serratus anterior

iliopsoas*

sartorius
pectineus*

adductor longus

gracilis*

Half Moon with Block

(Ardha Chandrasana)

Half Moon is a hip opener as well as a balancing posture. This version uses a block. With its rectangular shape, the block's sides give you three heights to choose from, depending on how limber you feel during your yoga practice.

1 Stand in Extended Triangle with Block (pages 36–37) with your right palm or fingertips on the block. Keep the alignment you found in Extended Triangle as you turn your gaze downward to your right foot. Bring your left hand onto your hip to help find your balance.

2 Bend your right knee slightly, keeping it extended over your middle toe as you move your block forward about a foot and a half in front of your right small toe. At the same time, shift more weight onto your right leg, and step your left foot in about 12 inches (30 cm).

3 Straighten your right leg, turning the thigh open clockwise while lifting your left leg parallel to

the floor to hip height or slightly higher. Keep your left leg in a neutral position, and flex your ankle.

4 Once you have your balance, extend your left arm straight up toward the ceiling, opening up across the front of your chest. Hold for 1 to 5 breaths.

5 To come out of the pose, bring your left hand onto your hip. Bend your right knee, keeping it over your middle toes as you step your left leg back about 3 or 4 feet (1 meter). Straighten your right leg, move the block, and transition back into Extended Triangle, then continue to reverse your steps back into Warrior II.

6 From Warrior II, follow either Transition 1 or Transition 2 (page 63) to end in Downward-Facing Dog. Then, repeat all steps on the left side. After doing both sides, move into Transition 4 (pages 63) to end in Mountain Pose.

Correct form
· Turn your gaze toward the floor, to the side, or up to your raised hand.
· To help activate your lifted leg, imagine that you are pressing your flexed foot into a wall behind you.

Avoid
· Letting your standing foot turn in.
· Allowing the knee of your standing foot to twist out of alignment.

Diary of practice

	Date	No. of Breaths	Comment
Week 1			
Week 2			
Week 3			
Week 4			

Annotation Key
* indicates deep muscles

tensor fasciae latae

obliquus externus

serratus anterior

rectus femoris

adductor longus

pectineus*

iliopsoas*

rectus abdominis

transversus abdominis*

obliquus internus*

vastus lateralis

vastus intermedius*

vastus medialis

Back View

gluteus medius*

gluteus maximus

quadratus femoris*

obdurator internus*

obdurator externus*

semitendinosus

biceps femoris

semimembranosus

Chair Pose
(Utkatasana)

Chair Pose is a versatile pose, because you can easily control its intensity, bending your knees just a few inches or all the way down so that your hips are in line with your knees. This pose is part of Sun Salutation B.

1 Begin in Mountain Pose (pages 24–25), with your feet together and arms by your sides. Inhale your arms into Upward Salute (pages 22–23), reaching above your head so that your arms are parallel to each other. Rotate your outer upper arms inward and reach up through your fingertips.

2 Exhale, and bend your knees. Both ankles, inner thighs, and knees should be touching. Bring your weight onto your heels, try to shift your hips back, and draw your knees right above your ankles. Hold for 1 to 5 breaths.

3 Straighten your legs and fold forward into Standing Forward Bend to begin the vinyasa, ending in Downward-Facing Dog (pages 16–17).

Correct form
· Find a neutral position by drawing your tailbone down as you roll your inner thighs toward the floor.

Avoid
· Over-tucking your pelvis.
· Over-arching your lower back.
· Letting your feet separate or your knees knock inward.
· Lifting your heels.

Diary of practice

	Date	No. of Breaths	Comment
Week 1			
Week 2			
Week 3			
Week 4			

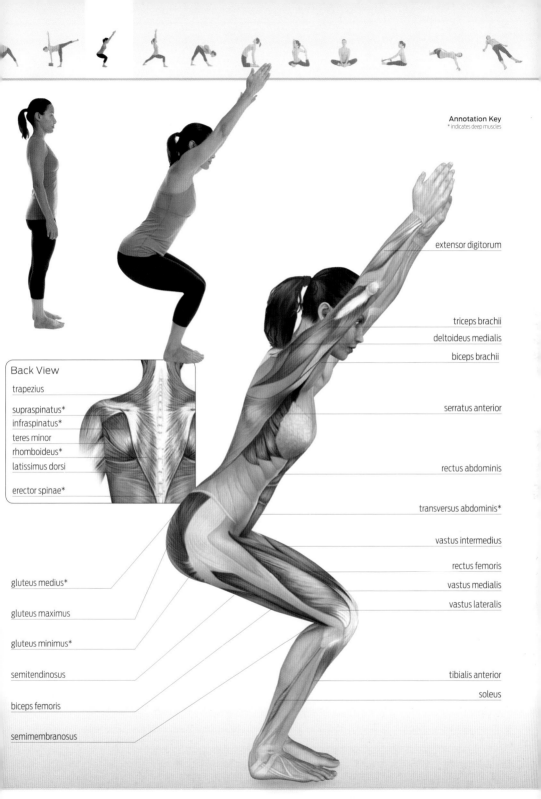

Annotation Key
* indicates deep muscles

extensor digitorum

triceps brachii
deltoideus medialis
biceps brachii

serratus anterior

rectus abdominis

transversus abdominis*

vastus intermedius

rectus femoris
vastus medialis
vastus lateralis

tibialis anterior
soleus

Back View

trapezius

supraspinatus*
infraspinatus*
teres minor
rhomboideus*
latissimus dorsi

erector spinae*

gluteus medius*

gluteus maximus

gluteus minimus*

semitendinosus

biceps femoris

semimembranosus

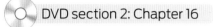

Warrior I
(Virabhadrasana I)

Warrior I requires a mix of fortitude and flexibility. With practice, you will build strength and increase your confidence both on and off the mat.

1 From Downward-Facing Dog (pages 16–17), step your right foot forward into High Lunge (pages 18–19), pivot your left heel down, and angle your left toes to face the upper left corner of your mat. Walk your right foot to the right several inches, so that your feet are in heel-to-heel alignment.

2 Keep your left leg straight and your right knee bent as you inhale, lifting your torso and arms above your head, with your body in a straight line. Externally rotate both arms, palms facing toward each other, and energy up through your fingertips.

3 Hold the pose for 1 to 5 breaths with your shoulders, torso, and hips squared to the front of the mat. Your bent knee should be in line with your middle toe. Aim to bend so that your thigh is parallel to the floor. Press into the outer edge of your left foot and firm your left thigh as you slightly internally rotate the leg.

4 To come out of the pose, place your hands on the floor and lift your left heel back into High Lunge. From High Lunge continue through the entire Sun Salutation B sequence (page 61), including the left side, to end in Mountain Pose (pages 24–25).

Diary of practice

	Date	No. of Breaths	Comment
Week 1			
Week 2			
Week 3			
Week 4			

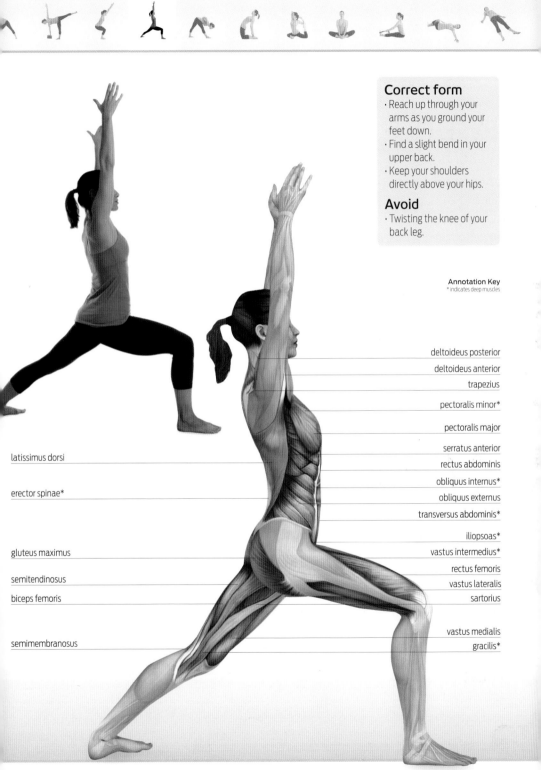

Correct form
· Reach up through your arms as you ground your feet down.
· Find a slight bend in your upper back.
· Keep your shoulders directly above your hips.

Avoid
· Twisting the knee of your back leg.

Annotation Key
* indicates deep muscles

deltoideus posterior

deltoideus anterior

trapezius

pectoralis minor*

pectoralis major

serratus anterior

latissimus dorsi

rectus abdominis

obliquus internus*

erector spinae*

obliquus externus

transversus abdominis*

iliopsoas*

gluteus maximus

vastus intermedius*

rectus femoris

semitendinosus

vastus lateralis

biceps femoris

sartorius

vastus medialis

semimembranosus

gracilis*

Intense Side Stretch

(Parsvottanasana)

Intense Side Stretch is a forward bend that is calming, while it also provides an intense stretch for your hamstrings—especially beneficial if you like to run.

1 From Mountain Pose (pages 24–25), step your left foot back about 3 feet (1 meter). Turn your toes in about 45 degrees so that they face the upper left corner of your mat. Come into heel-to-heel alignment, squaring your hips to the front of the mat.

2 Extend your arms out parallel to the floor, turn your thumbs down, bend your elbows, and join your hands into a prayer position: begin with the backs of your hands together and the fingers pointing down, and then turn your fingers away from your back and flip your wrists so that your fingers point upward. Press your pinky fingers together, and slowly try to press your hands together.

3 Inhale, broadening across your collar bones, drawing your shoulder blades together and lifting your chest while keeping your hips squared.

4 Ground through the pinky toe edge of your left foot, and press your left thigh back as you exhale to fold forward over your right leg. Lead with your heart and keep your spine elongated. Hold for 1 to 5 breaths.

5 Inhale, draw your shoulders back, and lift your sternum, leading with your heart to come up to standing. Step your left foot forward to meet your right foot in Mountain Pose, and repeat on the other side.

6 Repeat the first nine steps of Sun Salutation A (page 60), ending in Downward-Facing Dog (pages 16–17).

Correct form
· As you square your hips, draw your right hip crease back as you press your right big toe down to counteract that movement.
· If you have tight hamstrings, try widening your stance by walking your right foot closer to the right edge of the mat.

Avoid
· Rounding your back as you fold forward.

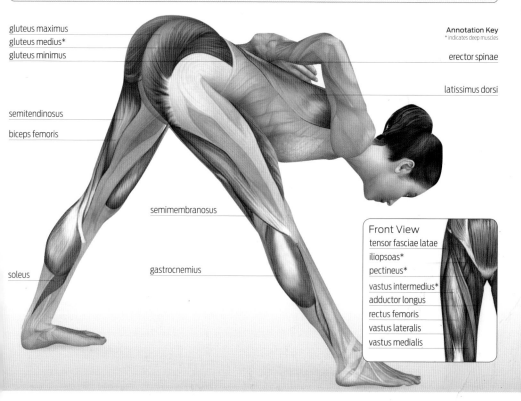

Diary of practice

	Date	No. of Breaths	Comment
Week 1			
Week 2			
Week 3			
Week 4			

gluteus maximus
gluteus medius*
gluteus minimus

semitendinosus

biceps femoris

semimembranosus

gastrocnemius

soleus

Annotation Key
* indicates deep muscles

erector spinae

latissimus dorsi

Front View
tensor fasciae latae
iliopsoas*
pectineus*
vastus intermedius*
adductor longus
rectus femoris
vastus lateralis
vastus medialis

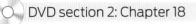

Camel Pose

(Ustrasana)

Camel Pose is a heart-opening backbend that stretches the shoulders and lower back.

1 From Downward-Facing Dog (pages 16–17), come into a kneeling position, with your knees hip-width apart and shins and feet aligned behind them. The tops of your feet should be on the floor, your toes pointing straight back.

2 Bend your elbows, and bring your hands to your lower back, fingers pointing upward. Draw your elbows together, opening your chest. Internally rotate your thighs, and use the heels of your palms to draw your buttocks toward the floor as you lift out of your lower back.

3 Bend from your upper back, and straighten your arms as you reach behind you to grasp your heels. Keep your hips directly above your knees; if your hips shift backward as you reach for your toes, then keep your hands on your lower back. With practice, you will eventually be able to bend back to reach your heels.

4 Broaden across your collarbones and press your shoulder blades in and up to open your chest and shoulders. Allow your head to drop back. Hold for 1 to 5 breaths.

5 To come out of the pose, exhale to lift your head and torso and sit into Child's Pose (pages 14–15), releasing your back. If desired, repeat Camel Pose 2 or 3 times, and then return to Downward-Facing Dog (pages 16–17).

Correct form
· While bending back, keep your thighs perpendicular to the floor.
· If your neck feels stressed when you drop your head back, just keep your head lifted, and gaze forward.

Avoid
· Bending from your hips.
· Arching your lower back.

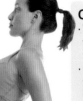

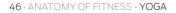

Diary of practice

	Date	No. of Breaths	Comment
Week 1			
Week 2			
Week 3			
Week 4			

sternocleidomastoideus

pectoralis major

rectus abdominis

pectoralis minor*

trapezius

deltoideus posterior

coracobrachialis*

triceps brachii

biceps brachii

gluteus maximus

semitendinosus

biceps femoris

semimembranosus

Annotation Key
* indicates deep muscles

Front View
tensor fasciae latae
iliopsoas*
pectineus*
vastus intermedius*
adductor longus
rectus femoris
vastus lateralis
vastus medialis

Pigeon Pose
(Eka Pada Rajakapotasana)

Pigeon Pose is a very challenging pose because it demands flexibility in the hips, thighs, spine, and shoulders.

1 From Downward-Facing Dog (pages 16–17), inhale and lift your right leg up behind you.

2 On an exhale, bend your right knee into your chest and then lower your body so that your right knee is on the floor in front of you, foot facing left, right shin and foot on the floor. Draw your right shin slightly forward, and flex your right ankle to keep your knee in alignment.

3 Extend your left leg behind you, with the top of your foot on the floor and toes pointing straight back.

4 Slowly lift your torso upright, bend your left knee, and hold onto your foot with your left hand. Lift up out of the lower back by drawing your tailbone down as you lift your pubic bone toward your frontal hipbones.

5 Bring your foot into the crook of your left elbow before reaching your right arm up, bending the elbow toward the ceiling, and clasping your hands as you continue to square the hips and shoulders. Hold for 1 to 5 breaths.

6 To come out of the pose, straighten your left leg and tuck your left toes under. Place your hands flat onto the floor, straighten your arms and place your right foot onto the floor into High Lunge (pages 18–19). Then step your right leg back into Downward-Facing Dog. Repeat on the other side.

Correct form
· Bend from your thoracic spine.
· Internally rotate your thigh to place your left leg behind you.
· If desired, place padding under your buttocks for support.
· You can place a block or a blanket under your right hip if there is space between your hip and the floor. Support your hips so that you can keep your sacrum level and help square the hips to the front of the mat.

Avoid
· Bending from your lumbar spine.

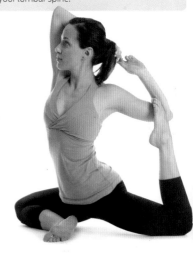

Diary of practice

	Date	No. of Breaths	Comment
Week 1			
Week 2			
Week 3			
Week 4			

Front View

tensor fasciae latae
iliopsoas*
pectineus*
vastus intermedius*
rectus femoris
vastus lateralis
vastus medialis

triceps brachii

Annotation Key
* indicates deep muscles

serratus anterior
rectus abdominis
obliquus externus
obliquus internus*
transversus abdominis*

adductor longus
adductor magnus

sternocleidomastoideus
rhomboideus*
pectoralis minor
pectoralis major
latissimus dorsi

erector spinae*

gluteus medius*
gluteus maximus
gluteus minimus*

biceps femoris

○ DVD section 2: Chapter 20

Bound Angle Pose
(Baddha Konasana)

Beneficial for all levels, Bound Angle Pose is a great hip opener. To execute this pose properly, aim your navel toward your feet—not your head.

1 From Pigeon Pose (48–49), swing your right leg around in front, shifting your weight onto the left hip.

2 Bend both knees and bring the soles of your feet together as you draw your feet in toward your pelvis, keeping your knees apart. Hold your ankles and press the small-toe side of both feet together, "opening" the insides of your feet as if you were opening a book.

3 Inhale as you lengthen your sternum and open your collarbones. Exhale, and fold forward, leading with your heart.

Correct form
· To make the pose feel more restorative, rest your forehead on a block.

Avoid
· Rounding your upper back to fold forward.
· Forcing your knees down.

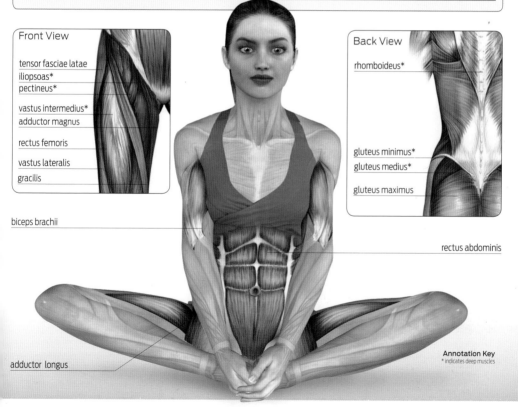

Diary of practice

	Date	No. of Breaths	Comment
Week 1			
Week 2			
Week 3			
Week 4			

Front View

tensor fasciae latae
iliopsoas*
pectineus*

vastus intermedius*
adductor magnus

rectus femoris

vastus lateralis

gracilis

biceps brachii

Back View

rhomboideus*

gluteus minimus*
gluteus medius*

gluteus maximus

rectus abdominis

adductor longus

Annotation Key
* indicates deep muscles

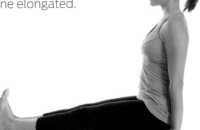

DVD section 2: Chapter 21

Seated Forward Bend
(Paschimottanasana)

Seated Forward Bend is an introspective posture. It requires you to "surrender," reducing stress and calming the mind. This version uses a yoga strap so that you can keep your spine elongated.

1 From Bound Angle Pose (pages 50–51) lift your knees with your hands until your feet are flat on the floor, and then straighten your legs in front of you with feet flexed. Firm your thighs into the floor.

2 Place your yoga strap under the balls of your feet so that the strap wraps around both feet. Inhale, lengthening your spine, and exhale to fold forward, "walking" your hands forward on the strap.

3 Hinge at your hips and bring your belly toward your thighs. Maintain a slight arch in your lower back as you root your thighs down toward the floor, which will help you to fold more deeply. Inhale to lengthen your spine and exhale to fold farther into your legs.

Correct form
- Lengthen from the base of your spine.
- Lead with your heart.
- Your feet should be straight, as if you were standing in Mountain Pose.

Avoid
- Rounding your upper back.

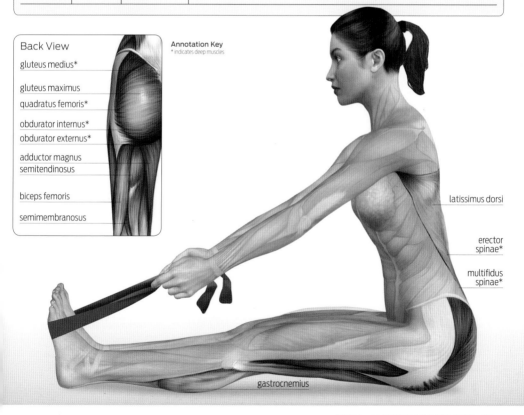

Diary of practice

	Date	No. of Breaths	Comment
Week 1			
Week 2			
Week 3			
Week 4			

Back View

gluteus medius*

gluteus maximus
quadratus femoris*

obdurator internus*
obdurator externus*

adductor magnus
semitendinosus

biceps femoris

semimembranosus

Annotation Key
* indicates deep muscles

latissimus dorsi

erector
spinae*

multifidus
spinae*

gastrocnemius

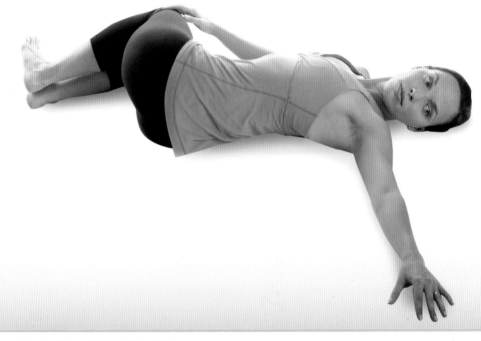

DVD section 2: Chapter 22

Reclining Twist
(Jathara Parivrrti)

Reclining Twist can be performed at any level. It is very relaxing, so you can practice it with your eyes closed before moving into Corpse Pose.

1 Lie on your back. Bend your knees into your chest and extend your arms into a T position with your palms facing downward.

2 Drop both of your knees to the right and hold onto them with your right hand. Twist your upper back around to the left. Turn your head to the left and either close your eyes or gaze toward your left fingertips. Hold for 1 to 5 breaths.

3 Return your knees to center, and then repeat the entire twist in the opposite direction.

Correct form
· Relax into the twist.
· Stack your legs one on top of the other so that the knees, shins, and ankles line up.
· For a deeper twist, lift both shoulders a couple of inches off the floor and then place them back down.

Avoid
· Raising your arms too high if you have shoulder pain.

Diary of practice

	Date	No. of Breaths	Comment
Week 1			
Week 2			
Week 3			
Week 4			

tractus iliotibialis

quadratus lumborum*

obliquus externus

gluteus maximus

gluteus medius*

serratus anterior

erector spinae*

obliquus internus*

rectus abdominis

pectoralis major

pectoralis minor*

scalenus*

sternocleidomastoideus

splenius*

levator scapulae*

Front View

tensor fasciae latae
iliopsoas*
pectineus*
vastus intermedius*
adductor longus

rectus femoris

vastus lateralis

Annotation Key
* indicates deep muscles

Corpse Pose
(Savasana)

Corpse Pose, commonly called Savasana, may look easy, but it can be highly challenging. It requires total "surrender" and quieting of the body and mind. Your goal is to let gravity—not your muscles—do the work for you.

1 Lie on your back, and let your arms release outward from your sides far enough from your body for your armpits to have space. Relax your hands and face your palms upward.

2 Let your legs separate to about as wide as your mat so that your lower back starts to release. Allow your legs, feet, and ankles to relax completely. Draw your buttocks down toward your heels to create length in your lower back; to help with this, you can lift your hips slightly and use your hands to draw your buttocks down away from your waist before you completely relax.

3 Let your eyes, jaw, tongue, and throat soften. Release any controlled breath, and begin to breathe quietly. Remain here for 3 to 10 minutes.

4 To transition out of Savasana, inhale and exhale deeply and then start to wiggle your fingers and toes, making small movements to bring awareness back to the rest of the body. Hug both knees into your chest, and then gently roll over onto your right side, taking pressure away from the heart. Pause there for a moment in a fetal position. Slowly press yourself up to sit in Easy Pose (pages 12–13), keeping your eyes closed. Stay there for several breaths (or minutes) before opening your eyes.

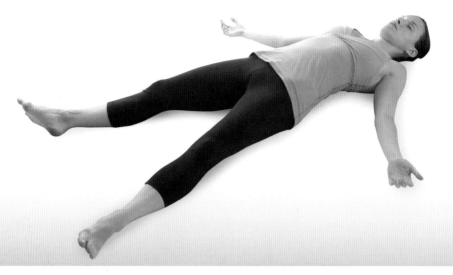

Diary of practice

	Date	No. of Breaths	Comment
Week 1			
Week 2			
Week 3			
Week 4			

Correct form
· Place a rolled-up blanket underneath your knees if you feel any lower-back discomfort.
· Make sure that your body isn't touching anything near your mat, such as your block, strap, or water bottle.

Avoid
· Keeping your eyes open and letting them wander around the room.
· Positioning your body asymmetrically.

Full-Body Anatomy

scalenus*

pectoralis major

deltoideus anterior

coracobrachialis*

rectus abdominis

obliquus externus

palmaris longus

flexor carpi ulnaris

flexor carpi radialis

transversus abdominis*

sartorius

vastus intermedius*

rectus femoris

vastus lateralis

vastus medialis

tibialis anterior

peroneus

extensor hallucis

adductor hallucis

sternocleidomastoideus

pectoralis minor*

biceps brachii

serratus anterior

obliquus internus*

pronator teres

flexor digitorum*

extensor carpi radialis

flexor carpi pollicis longus

tensor fasciae latae

iliopsoas*

iliacus*

pectineus*

adductor longus

gracilis*

gastrocnemius

soleus

flexor digitorum

extensor digitorum

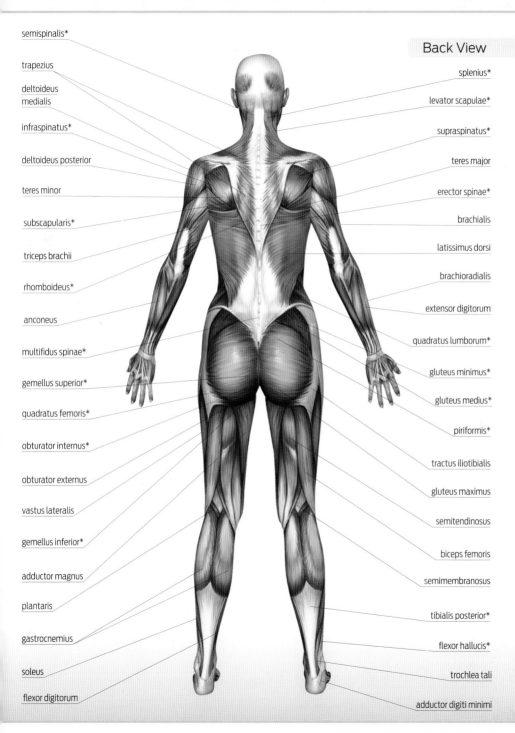

semispinalis*

trapezius

deltoideus
medialis

infraspinatus*

deltoideus posterior

teres minor

subscapularis*

triceps brachii

rhomboideus*

anconeus

multifidus spinae*

gemellus superior*

quadratus femoris*

obturator internus*

obturator externus

vastus lateralis

gemellus inferior*

adductor magnus

plantaris

gastrocnemius

soleus

flexor digitorum

splenius*

levator scapulae*

supraspinatus*

teres major

erector spinae*

brachialis

latissimus dorsi

brachioradialis

extensor digitorum

quadratus lumborum*

gluteus minimus*

gluteus medius*

piriformis*

tractus iliotibialis

gluteus maximus

semitendinosus

biceps femoris

semimembranosus

tibialis posterior*

flexor hallucis*

trochlea tali

adductor digiti minimi

The Sun Salutations

Sun Salutation A
Sun Salutation A can be performed 2 to 5 times to build heat.

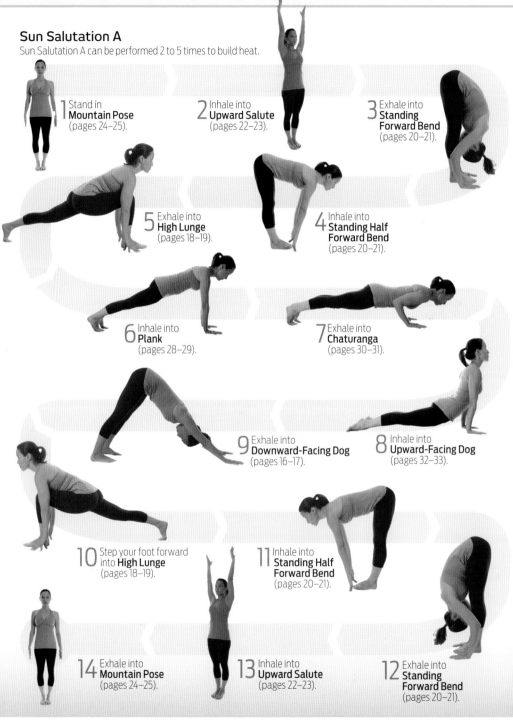

1 Stand in **Mountain Pose** (pages 24–25).

2 Inhale into **Upward Salute** (pages 22–23).

3 Exhale into **Standing Forward Bend** (pages 20–21).

4 Inhale into **Standing Half Forward Bend** (pages 20–21).

5 Exhale into **High Lunge** (pages 18–19).

6 Inhale into **Plank** (pages 28–29).

7 Exhale into **Chaturanga** (pages 30–31).

8 Inhale into **Upward-Facing Dog** (pages 32–33).

9 Exhale into **Downward-Facing Dog** (pages 16–17).

10 Step your foot forward into **High Lunge** (pages 18–19).

11 Inhale into **Standing Half Forward Bend** (pages 20–21).

12 Exhale into **Standing Forward Bend** (pages 20–21).

13 Inhale into **Upward Salute** (pages 22–23).

14 Exhale into **Mountain Pose** (pages 24–25).

Sun Salutation B

Sun Salutation B can be performed 2 to 5 times to build heat.

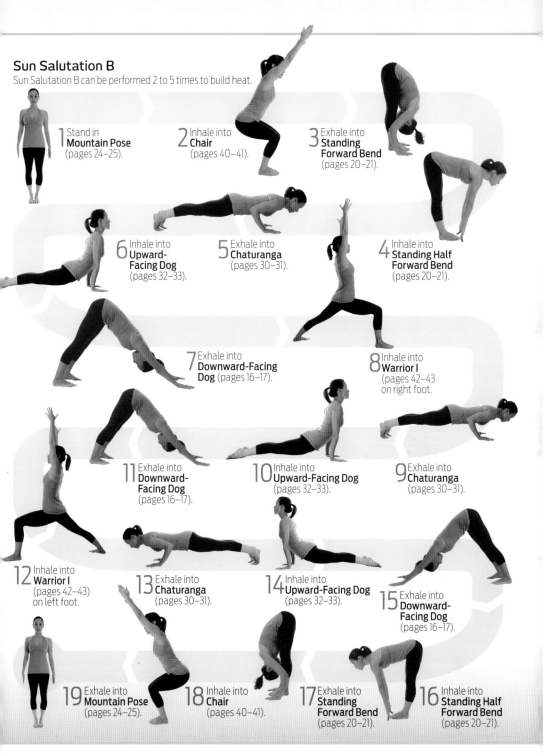

1 Stand in **Mountain Pose** (pages 24–25).

2 Inhale into **Chair** (pages 40–41).

3 Exhale into **Standing Forward Bend** (pages 20–21).

4 Inhale into **Standing Half Forward Bend** (pages 20–21).

5 Exhale into **Chaturanga** (pages 30–31).

6 Inhale into **Upward-Facing Dog** (pages 32–33).

7 Exhale into **Downward-Facing Dog** (pages 16–17).

8 Inhale into **Warrior I** (pages 42–43 on right foot.

9 Exhale into **Chaturanga** (pages 30–31).

10 Inhale into **Upward-Facing Dog** (pages 32–33).

11 Exhale into **Downward-Facing Dog** (pages 16–17).

12 Inhale into **Warrior I** (pages 42–43) on left foot.

13 Exhale into **Chaturanga** (pages 30–31).

14 Inhale into **Upward-Facing Dog** (pages 32–33).

15 Exhale into **Downward-Facing Dog** (pages 16–17).

16 Inhale into **Standing Half Forward Bend** (pages 20–21).

17 Exhale into **Standing Forward Bend** (pages 20–21).

18 Inhale into **Chair** (pages 40–41).

19 Exhale into **Mountain Pose** (pages 24–25).

Vinyasa & Other Transitions

Vinyasa

The vinyasa is a sequence that you will repeat several times during your yoga practice to transition between sustained poses performed to the left or the right. As you become more adept, you will begin to smoothly flow through these movements.

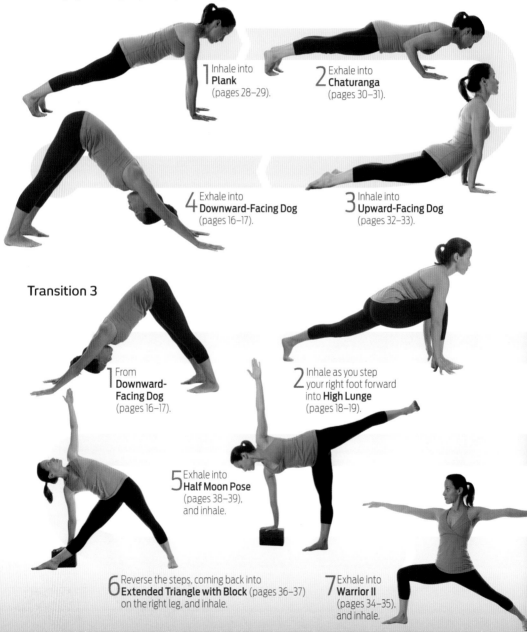

1 Inhale into **Plank** (pages 28–29).

2 Exhale into **Chaturanga** (pages 30–31).

3 Inhale into **Upward-Facing Dog** (pages 32–33).

4 Exhale into **Downward-Facing Dog** (pages 16–17).

Transition 3

1 From **Downward-Facing Dog** (pages 16–17).

2 Inhale as you step your right foot forward into **High Lunge** (pages 18–19).

5 Exhale into **Half Moon Pose** (pages 38–39), and inhale.

6 Reverse the steps, coming back into **Extended Triangle with Block** (pages 36–37) on the right leg, and inhale.

7 Exhale into **Warrior II** (pages 34–35), and inhale.

Other important transitions

You will repeat these sequences throughout your yoga practice.

Transition 1
· Inhale from **Warrior II** (pages 34–35).
· Move into **Plank** (pages 28–29).
· Exhale to **Downward-Facing Dog** (pages 16–17).

Transition 2
· From **Warrior II** (pages 34–35), inhale to begin the **vinyasa** (see opposite), ending in **Downward-Facing Dog** (pages 16–17).

Transition 3 (pictured below)
· From **Downward-Facing Dog** (pages 16–17), inhale as you step your right foot forward into **High Lunge** (pages 18–19).
· Pivot your left heel down, exhale and come into **Warrior II** (pages 34–35), and inhale.
· Exhale into **Extended Triangle with Block** (pages 36–37) on the right leg, and inhale.

· Exhale into **Half Moon Pose with Block** (pages 38–39), and inhale.
· Reverse the steps, coming back into **Extended Triangle with Block** (pages 36–37) on the right leg, and inhale.
· Exhale into **Warrior II** (pages 34–35), and inhale.
· Exhale into **High Lunge** (pages 18–19), and inhale.
· Exhale to **Downward-Facing Dog** (pages 16–17).

Transition 4
· From **Downward-Facing Dog** (pages 16–17) step into **High Lunge** (pages 18–19), then come to the front of your mat.
· Inhale, and lengthen the spine into **Standing Half Forward Bend** (pages 20–21).
· Exhale to **Standing Forward Bend** (pages 20–21).
· Inhale to **Upward Salute** (pages 22–23).
· Exhale to **Mountain Pose** (pages 24–25).

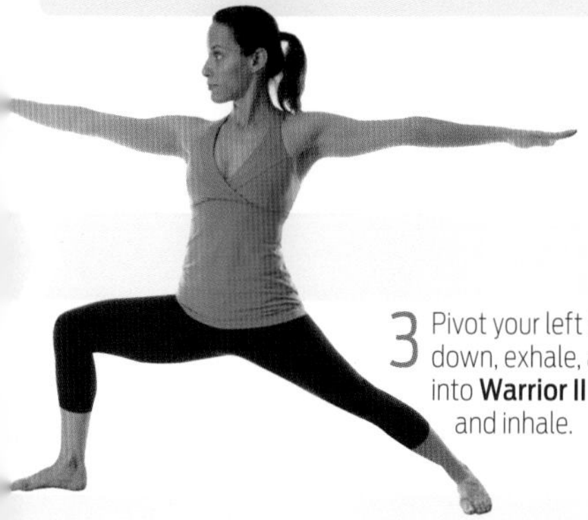

3 Pivot your left heel down, exhale, and come into **Warrior II** (pages 34–35), and inhale.

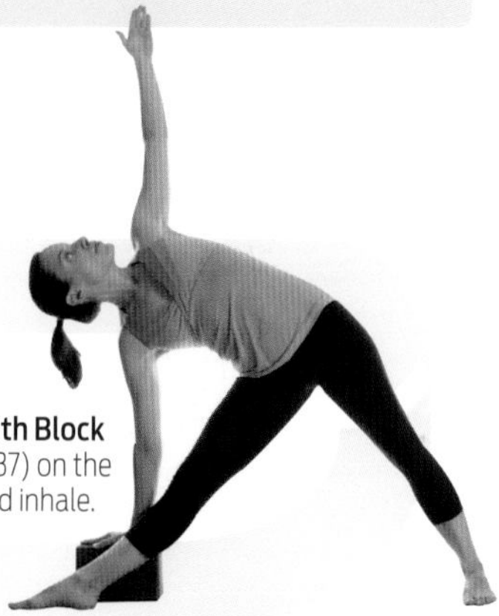

4 Exhale into **Extended Triangle with Block** (pages 36–37) on the right leg, and inhale.

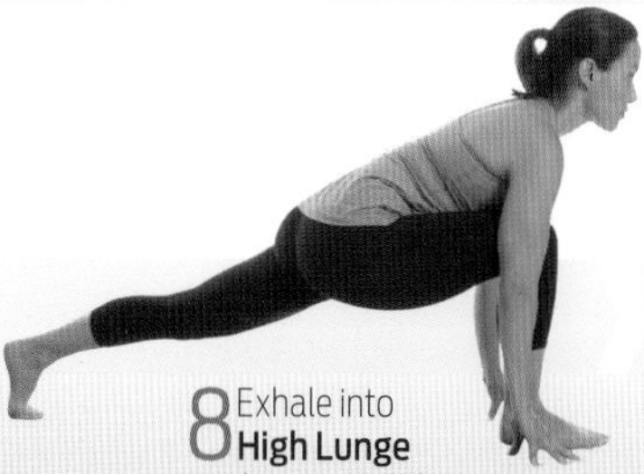

8 Exhale into **High Lunge** (pages 18–19), and inhale.

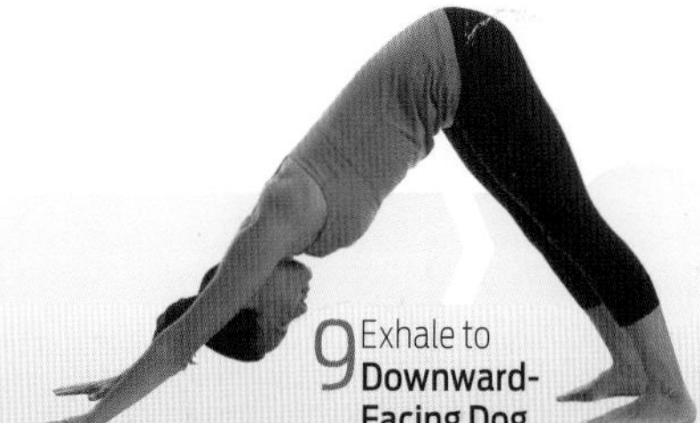

9 Exhale to **Downward-Facing Dog** (pages 16–17).

About the Author

Goldie Karpel Oren began ballet training at the age of three and continued training through high school. During high school she performed with Dances Patrelle in New York as well as Ballet Rox in Boston. She received a B.A from Johns Hopkins University, Baltimore, in 2006, with a major in creative writing. After graduating from college she was a soloist with the Atlantic City Ballet. In spring 2008, Goldie developed an injury that forced her to stop dancing but led her to yoga, which became another passion. Goldie studied yoga and became RYT certified. She now teaches yoga at several studios and works individually with private clients in their homes in New York City. This is Goldie's first published work.

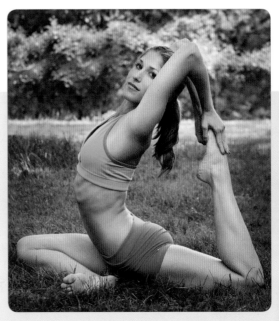

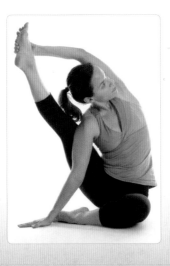

Yoga model Lana Russo is a 500-hour registered yoga teacher with the Yoga Alliance. She earned her training through the Long Island Yoga School in New York and is currently a teacher trainer there, helping others on their journey toward teaching yoga. Lana teaches at many studios throughout the Long Island area and is a current yoga ambassador for Lululemon Athletica. As a former ballet dancer, she enjoys the flow of vinyasa yoga and loves to help bring students to their own personal edge. In her spare time, she enjoys being with her husband and daughter.